THE ESSENTIAL HANDBOOK TO A HEALTHY GUT

HOW A LEAKY GUT IMPACTS

YOUR ENTIRE BODY AND HOW

TO MAKE IT HEALTHY ONCE AGAIN

BY

EVELYN CARMICHAEL

Copyright © 2017

Evelyn Carmichael

INTRODUCTION

Is your gut impacting your health? Find out if your gut is responsible for inflammation and a host of medical issues from anxiety to autoimmune disorders.

If you have an unhealthy gut, chances are you frequently suffer from heartburn, constipation, bloating, abdominal pain and diarrhea. These symptoms occur frequently in people who have gut issues. But the good news is they can all be treated.

Many people tend to treat the symptoms of an unhealthy gut, rather than trying to boost the health of the gut in the first place. While there is nothing wrong with this, if you don't treat the root cause of the issue, it's likely that you will be experiencing those symptoms again and again. Medication that can help to treat the symptoms of a leaky gut may actually be making your gut even more unhealthy.

In this book, you will find out how to improve the health of your gut. Specifically, we will look at:

- What is Leaky Gut?
- How your gut can impact your entire health, including triggering inflammation throughout your body that may cause autoimmune disorders, mood disorders, heart attacks, and cancer.
- How food intolerances and allergies play a role including gluten and lectins.
- How stress and medications impact your gut
- How fiber can repair your gut
- Pre and Probiotics
- How what you eat can heal your gut

This Essential Handbook will give you a beginning guide on how you can make significant changes to your gut health and improve your overall well-being.

The Essential Handbook to a Healthy Gut

Evelyn Carmichael

TABLE OF CONTENTS

Evelyn Carmichael

LEGAL NOTES

Disclaimer: All content of this handbook is created for educational and informational purposes. This author is not affiliated with any specific diet plan, medical treatment, pharmaceutical or holistic company. Before any change of diet or medication, it is recommended to consult your physician. Personal use of any content is to be taken at the sole risk of the individual. The author and publisher bare no responsibility therein.

The Essential Handbook to a Healthy Gut

Evelyn Carmichael

CHAPTER 1. WHY IS GUT HEALTH SO IMPORTANT?

Most of us are unaware of just how important it is to have a healthy gut. We assume that eating a healthy diet, and getting enough exercise is sufficient, but this is not always the case.

Hippocrates is quoted as saying "All disease begins in the gut", and to a degree he was right. Your gut is the largest immune system organ in your body. When your gut, also known as your gastrointestinal system, is not as healthy as it could be, your immune system is likely to suffer, and you could start to become more susceptible to colds and sinus conditions.

Having a healthy gut can impact the health of your entire body. When your gut is healthy, you will not only have better digestion but also an improved mood and better overall health. With this is mind it's easy to see why gut health is so important.

What is a Leaky Gut?

When discussing gut health, you may have heard of a Leaky Gut or Intestinal Permeability. When your small intestine becomes damaged, small food particles and bacteria leak into your bloodstream. In fact, this isn't a medical diagnosis, but what one refers to for a wide range of symptoms impacting your intestine and your overall health. Gas, bloating, diarrhea, constipation, and pain are the most typically thought of symptoms, and those alone can cause a significant impact to your daily life. However, having a leaky gut can also impact your brain including problems with anxiety, depression, ADHD, memory, brain "fog", and headaches. Nutritional deficiencies may be found as well due to your body not properly digesting and absorbing the nutrients of the food you eat. There also may be overall issues with fatigue and aches and pains in your joints. Even your skin may be affected, with eczema, psoriasis, and acne symptoms.

A leaky gut can cause inflammation throughout your entire body as well as food intolerances. It can also trigger autoimmune diseases such as Chron's, Celiac Disease, Hashimoto's, Rheumatoid Arthritis, and Lupus.

Evelyn Carmichael

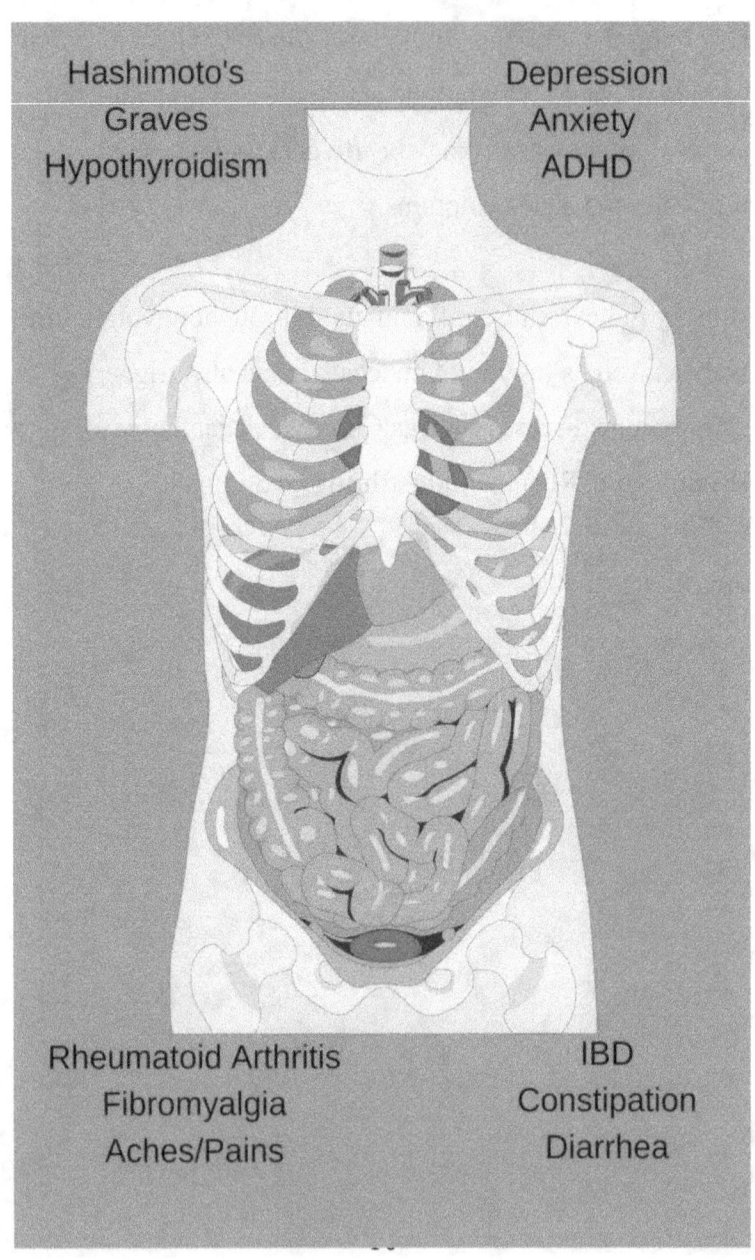

Hashimoto's   Depression
Graves   Anxiety
Hypothyroidism   ADHD

Rheumatoid Arthritis   IBD
Fibromyalgia   Constipation
Aches/Pains   Diarrhea

The Essential Handbook to a Healthy Gut

Evelyn Carmichael

CHAPTER 2. CAUSES OF A LEAKY GUT

There are several causes to a leaky gut. As depicted in the chart below, stress, food allergies, medications and other toxins, and bacteria are the main culprits. Many of us enjoy eating a wide range of foods, but most of us eat too much salt, sugar and fat that can often be hidden in processed foods. These foods can contribute to bad gut health, which means the gut will not work as effectively as it possibly could. When the gut is less efficient than it could be, food is not digested properly, which means the nutrients you consume may not benefit you as much as they possibly could. But food is only one part of the puzzle. For women, another cause for leaky gut can be hormonal imbalances caused by menstruation, pregnancy, or menopause. Let's take a closer look at some of the main culprits:

Evelyn Carmichael

LEAKY GUT PROGRESSION

STRESS **ALLERGIES** **MEDICATION TOXINS** **BACTERIA**

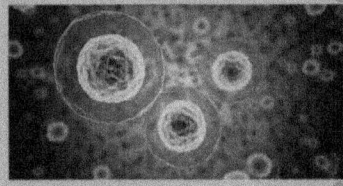

INTESTINAL CELLS

BLOOD STREAM

INFLAMMATION

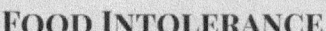

FOOD INTOLERANCE

AUTOIMMUNE DISEASE

Lectin and the Gluten Connection

Lectins are found in nearly all living organisms from plant roots to cow's milk. They are a carbohydrate-binding protein that attaches to cell membranes in order to communicate with the environment. Lectins are basically a toxin that is trying to communicate to its prey not to eat them. There are thousands of types of lectins, but 13 main classifications have emerged in the limited amount of research that has been conducted. Two types of lectins, agglutinins and prolamins appear to cause the most damage to the human body and are found in high lectin food.

Gluten is a type of lectin, belonging to the prolamin classification. So, when an individual cuts gluten out of their diet, they may only be cutting out part of the problem. If they have other lectin intolerances, they will continue to experience symptoms.

When your intestinal wall is permeated or damaged by lectins, the protein leaks out into your bloodstream. While in your bloodstream, the lectin binds to the surface of healthy cells and antibodies throughout your body. Your body sees this as an alien invasion and goes to work at attacking those cells. That attack is known as an autoimmune response. When this happens repeatedly, over time, your body can develop an autoimmune disease. The New England Journal of Medicine has listed 55 known diseases associated with gluten intolerance alone.

It is important to note that with lectin, a completely lectin-free diet is near impossible. The goal is to have a lower lectin diet for your gut to heal. But how can you improve the health of your gut? We are going to take a look at this in the next chapter.

The Essential Handbook to a Healthy Gut

Evelyn Carmichael

CHAPTER 3. HOW TO IMPROVE THE HEALTH OF YOUR GUT

In the last chapter, we saw that having an unhealthy gut can make you feel quite ill, and it could be one of the reasons why you feel tired and lethargic all the time. If the health of your gut is good, you will feel happier, you'll probably sleep better, and you'll have fewer colds too.

There are certain specific things you can do to improve your gut health. The chart on the next page depicts the nine most beneficial ways, though it is important to remember that the cause for poor gut health may vary from person to person and what makes one gut healthy may not work for another person. The items listed are an introduction to basic gut health. We will go into more detail on the most significant items in the upcoming chapters.

Evelyn Carmichael

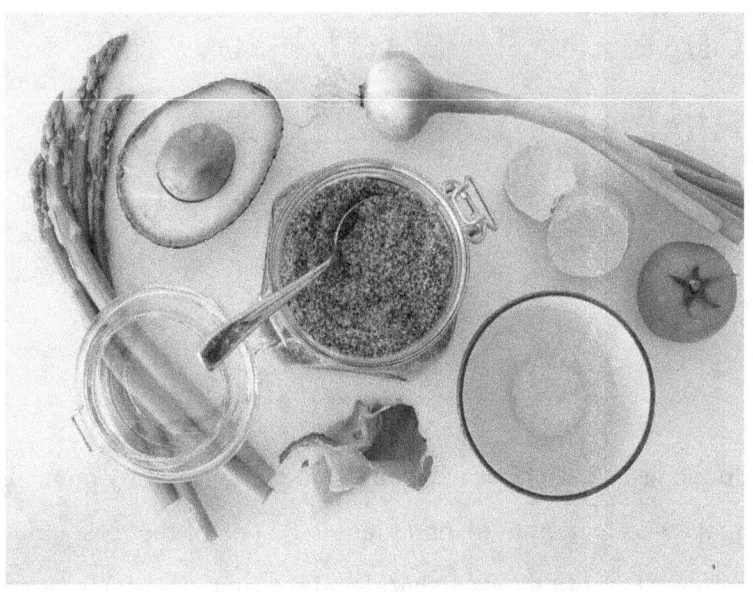

Top Nine Ways to Boost Gut Health

1. Add More Fiber/ Prebiotic Foods
2. Add Anti-Inflammatory Foods/ Spices
3. Add Fermented Foods
4. Decrease "Bad Gut" Foods
5. Avoid Prescription Drug Overuse
6. Reduce Stress
7. Reduce Sugar
8. Add a Probiotic
9. Examine Gut Allergies

So how can you improve the health of your gut?

It's thought that changing the way that you eat can have a huge effect on your gut health. This is good to know, because it's something all of us can do, without too much effort. Ok, so we all get used to eating the same foods now and again, but a few gradual changes here and there will really make a difference.

Did you know that making dietary changes can repair any damage that you have done to your gut? Similarly taking a few probiotic supplements can also help repair and prevent future damage.

Not everyone that has gut issues has a bad diet. Some people naturally have some sort of imbalance or food allergies, but this too can be improved. Let's dive deeper into some of the main gut health culprits and how to improve your gut.

Evelyn Carmichael

CHAPTER 4. DETERMINE ANY ALLERGIES/ INTOLERANCES

You may have noted that health articles, doctors, nutritionists, and even this book give conflicting advice on what to eat to improve gut health. Your friend may be loading up on high fiber legumes while you are on a strict low lectin (including gluten-free) diet. This is because the causes for an unhealthy gut vary and the treatment plan may be radically different from one person to the next. Unfortunately, finding out if you have allergies, or intolerances, is not the easiest thing to do. Speaking to your physician about the latest tests is a good first step. There are some blood tests and more invasive tests to determine if you have an intolerance. Remember, there are thousands of lectins out there, gluten being just one of them. Gluten itself is made up of hundreds of peptides and testing only measures a small fraction. The protein component of gluten is called gliadin and is made up of four sub classifications. The trouble is, most antibody testing only measures for one of the sub classifications, alpha. This leads to false negatives and individuals who have a gluten allergy to continue to eat gluten.

Here are some of the most current antibody testing your doctor may order:

- IgG anti-gliadin antibodies
- Total serum IgA antibodies
- tTg-IgA Tissue Transglutaminase antibodies
- IgA anti-gliadin antibodies
- IgA anti-endomysial antibodies
- Genetic testing (HLA DQ2 and HLA DQ8)
- Intestinal biopsy

Many physicians subscribe to the gluten elimination test. If you feel better after 30 days with a 100% gluten-free diet, then stick with that. A gluten-free diet may not be the only step you need to take. If you experienced a lessening of symptoms after undertaking a gluten-free diet but still have some lingering ills, you may want to reduce some of your higher lectin foods for lower lectin foods.

Evelyn Carmichael

CHAPTER 5. THE IMPORTANCE OF FIBER

Whether you have a gluten and/or lectin intolerance or not, fiber plays a significant role at improving gut health. Fiber is a carbohydrate that is found in whole grains, fruits, beans, and vegetables. Unlike the rest of the carbohydrates that we eat, fiber is not easy for your body to digest. Here's where the gut comes in and assists in the digestion process. This fiber is digested by some of the good bacteria that lives in your gut, and once it has been digested, the bacteria starts to grow. This means you feel fuller longer, your blood sugar does not spike and the microbes in your gut have something to feed off of. Eating more of these foods can help your gut, and therefore help you feel so much better.

Researchers have been examining the role of fiber in your diet. A University of Michigan study looked at mice who had a high fiber diet. They had a healthy gut lining. Mice that were on a no-fiber diet had a permeable mucus (gut) lining, meaning that damage to the intestinal tract was allowing food and bacteria to leak from the gut lining. A third group of mice included mice that alternated between eating a high fiber diet one day and then a no-fiber diet the following day. Not surprising, the high-fiber days did not give enough protection to the gut. The mucus lining was roughly half the permeability as it should be. As a side benefit, the mice on the high- fiber diet consumed less calories than the other two groups and were slimmer. This is true of many studies that have shown that a high fiber diet can benefit your waistline as well as your gut lining!

How much fiber do I need?

Most individuals are eating about 15 grams of fiber a day. Our caveman ancestors are estimated to have eaten roughly

10 times that amount per day. The recommended daily amount is 25grams per day. Those with diabetes who are using fiber to help control insulin levels are often recommended 50grams of fiber per day. To lose weight, over 30 grams of fiber is recommended.

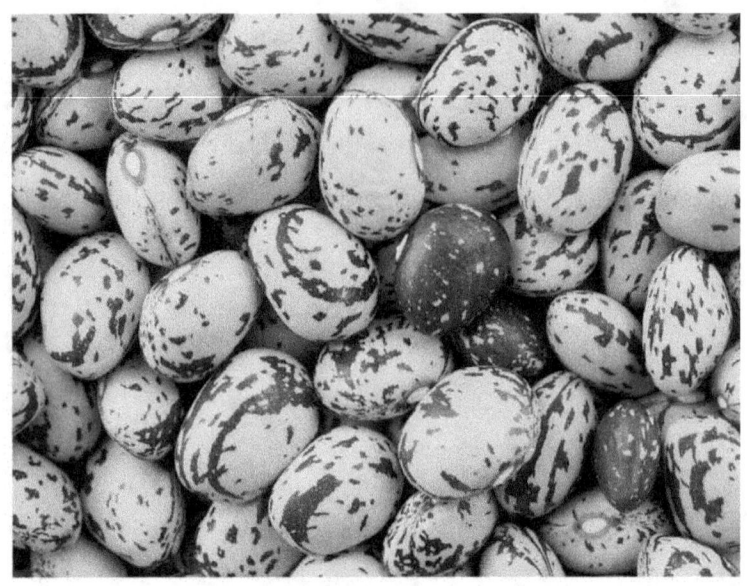

Top High Fiber Foods

Grain	Serving	Fiber (g)
Whole Wheat Flour	1 cup	13g
Quinoa(cooked)	1 cup	12g
Bran Cereal	½ cup	10g
Black Beans	1/2 cup	8g
Pinto Bean	1/2 cup	8g
Borlotti	1/2 cup	24g
Soybeans	1/2 cup	8g
Peanuts, dry-roast	1/2 cup	6g
Peas	1 cup	7g
Lentils	1/2 cup	8g
Chickpeas	1/2 cup	16g

Eating a balanced diet full of healthy fiber rich foods is recommended. Of course, those with a gluten intolerance should still be incorporating fiber in their diet. We will discuss gluten-free high fiber foods in more detail at the end of this chapter.

What you should eat

Ideally you should start to eat a wider range of foods. You may already eat a good mixture of foods, but adding more can certainly help. The idea is that you eat more fruits, vegetables, beans, and legumes, because these foods contain one of the best sources of microbiota, which is the new name for what used to be known as 'Gut flora'.

Microbiota is a term used to describe all the microbes that live in our gut, and they are responsible for helping your body to digest all your food. Some of the food that you consume cannot be easily digested by the small intestine or the stomach, and your gut goes to work to aid in digestion.

In addition to eating fruits, vegetables, beans, and legumes, you should also consume prebiotics, and these are foods that help to promote the development and growth of microbes in your gut. The microbes that prebiotics help to produce are beneficial ones which can contribute to the health of your gut.

Fruits, vegetables, beans, and legumes

I'm not suggesting that you only eat fruits, vegetables, beans, and legumes, I'm suggesting that you add more of them to your diet. These foods are one of the very best sources of microbiota, and we've already established that microbiota live in your gut, and they are responsible for helping your body to digest all your food.

Fruits, vegetables, beans, and legumes are also high in fiber, as well as other nutrients that your body needs. There are some foods that can really help you to improve your gut health, these foods could be considered 'Super foods', in that they are very high in fiber and can boost gut health:

- ✓ Artichokes

- ✓ Broccoli

- ✓ Chick peas

- ✓ Kidney beans

- ✓ Pinto beans

- ✓ Raspberries

- ✓ White beans

If you can, try to add more fruits, vegetables, beans, and legumes to your diet, while ensuring you get a higher intake of the 'Super foods' listed above.

Add anti-inflammatory foods and spices to your diet

Inflammation is your body fighting off what it believes to be a foreign substance. When you have a leaky gut, your body can become inflamed anywhere your gut particles have stuck to an otherwise healthy cell. When the cell becomes inflamed, your body is attacking the good healthy material underneath as well as the foreign substance. Chronic inflammation has been linked to autoimmune diseases as well as heart attacks, stroke, cancer, and arthritis, depression, and even Alzheimer's. Consuming foods that are anti-inflammatory in nature will help lessen inflammation in conjunction with the other techniques in this handbook. Below is a list of some foods that are particularly useful, though certainly not exhaustive, of anti-inflammatory foods and spices.

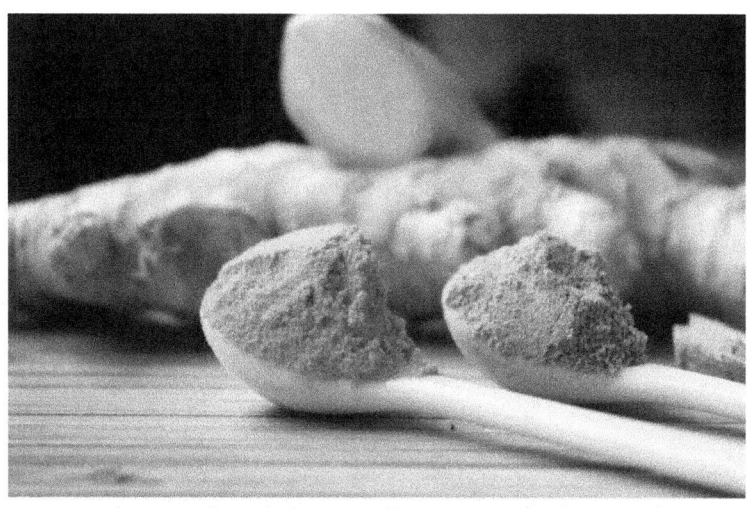

Top Anti-Inflammatory Foods & Spices

1. **Turmeric**
2. **Ginger**
3. **Green Leafy Vegetables**
4. **Green Tea**
5. **Dark Chocolate**
6. **Salmon**
7. **Chia Seeds**
8. **Blueberries**
9. **Broccoli**
10. **Garlic**
11. **Bok Choy**

Eat more whole grains

We are all encouraged to eat more whole grains, simply because they are very good for you, but not a lot of people are aware that whole grain foods can also contain a lot of gut-beneficial nutrients. This is because grains are digested in the large intestine and causes an increase in the healthy microbiota. A study in The Journal for Clinical Nutrition showed that whole grains increased heathy gut microbiota and reduced inflammation.

Below is a list of some whole grains that are very beneficial to adding fiber to your diet:

- ✓ Buckwheat – This whole grain can be enjoyed by those who can't eat gluten. But did you know that it's also tasty, and highly nutritive? Enjoy buckwheat in bread, pancakes, or sprinkled on a salad.

- ✓ Brown rice – Many people are happy to eat white rice, but did you know that brown rice contains a lot more nutrients? If you have the choice, you should choose brown rice instead of white. Just so you know, jasmine and basmati rice are brown, so you can enjoy them too, should you wish.

✓ Corn (Whole) – Corn is thought to be very good for you when you eat it whole. I know there are a lot of corn snacks out there, but these really aren't as healthy as completely unprocessed corn is. You may be pleased to know that you can eat popcorn, just make sure that it isn't completely covered in salt or sugar. Popping the corn yourself is a lot of fun, and with just a little bit of garlic or cinnamon sprinkled on it, it could be a really healthy snack.

✓ Oats (Whole) – We already know that oats contain prebiotics, but if you really want to benefit from the nutrients found in oats, you should try to eat them whole. If you're not a fan of eating porridge, try sprinkling some whole oats on some yogurt, or have them in or on top of a smoothie.

✓ Quinoa – Quinoa might not be a grain, but it's thought that this seed contains a lot more protein than any grain out there. This versatile food can be enjoyed in a wide variety of ways, helping you to benefit from its nutrients, and get that gut feeling great!

✓ Rye (Whole) – Rye in its natural form is thought to contain more nutrients than any other whole grain food. Incredibly, rye contains half of the iron you need, more fiber than whole wheat, and it's tasty too. When you're shopping for foods that contain rye, take a look at the ingredients list, and look for 'Whole rye'.

✓ Whole wheat – Whole wheat can be found in many pasta products, and in bread too. Beware that some foods will be marketed as being whole wheat, but they may simply contain regular wheat, or be a multigrain product. You need to be on the lookout for products that are 100% whole wheat, to be certain that you're getting the benefits.

Whole grain foods don't just contain a lot of fiber, they also contain a lot of gut-beneficial nutrients too. If you can add a little more whole grain to your day, you will soon start to see, and feel the benefits. Remember, whole grain foods don't have to tasty dull or boring, they can taste great, it's just up to you to make them taste that way. Experiment with whole grains and see what they can do for you.

Gluten Intolerance

There are plenty of high fiber foods for those who have a gluten intolerance. In fact, it is recommended that to improve gut health, a high fiber diet is just as important for those who cannot have many of the whole grains that are high in fiber.   The last section listed a couple of whole grain gluten-free foods, and below you will also find a list of high fiber gluten-free foods.

Evelyn Carmichael

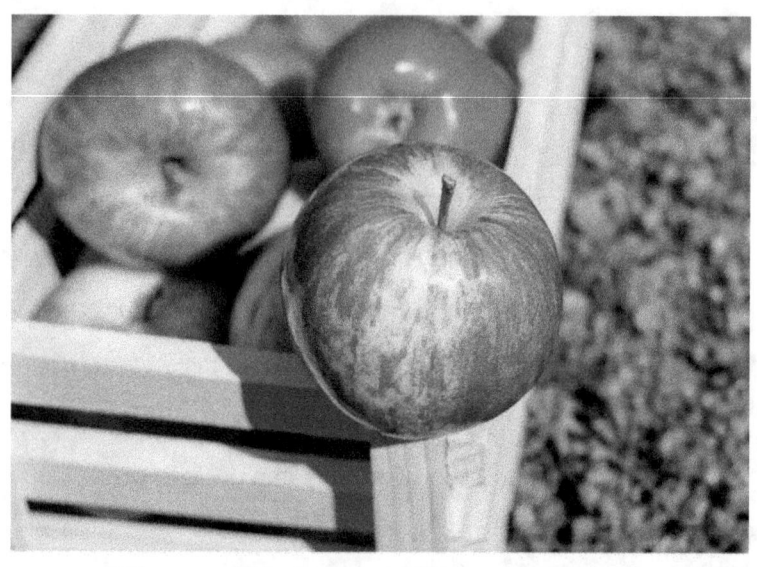

Top Gluten-Free High Fiber Foods

1. Almonds/ Almond Flour 3./5oz of fiber
2. Broccoli, Artichokes   4 grams/ cup
3. Apples, Pears (medium)   5 grams
4. Dark Chocolate   2 grams/oz.
5. Chickpeas   11 grams/cup
6. Buckwheat   4 grams/ 1/4 cup
7. Sweet Potatoes, Yams   5 grams/ cup
8. Raspberries   8 grams/ cup
9. Gluten-Free Oats   5 grams/ 1/4 cup
10. Kale   3 grams/ 1/2 cup

Lectin Intolerance

For those of you who are choosing lower lectin foods, you too can also have high fiber foods be a staple in your diet. Two areas to be of special concern are foods in the nightshade family and legumes. Both these categories are known for their high lectin foods. There are ways to make legumes lower in lectin. Specifically, by boiling, fermenting, or soaking legumes will help to naturally reduce the amount of lectin. Below you will find a chart of high fiber lower lectin foods.

Evelyn Carmichael

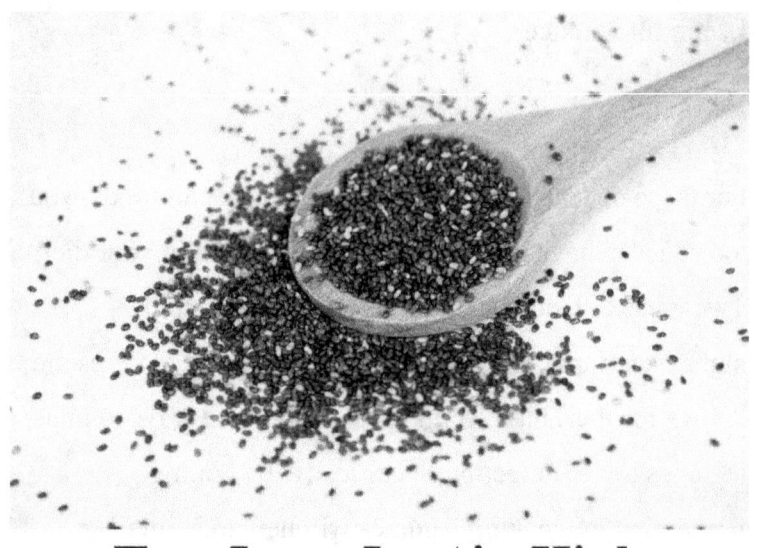

Top Low- Lectin High Fiber Foods

1 .Chia Seeds   10 grams/ oz. of fiber
2. Broccoli   4 grams/ cup
3. Apples, Pears (medium)   5 grams
4. Raspberries   8 grams/ cup
5. Cauliflower   5 grams/ cup
6. Kale   3 grams/ 1/2 cup
7. Walnuts   5 gram/ cup
8. Pecans   10 grams/ cup
9. Avocado   10 grams/ cup
10. Banana (medium)   3 grams

The Essential Handbook to a Healthy Gut

Evelyn Carmichael

CHAPTER 6. PREBIOTIC FOODS

Prebiotic foods are foods that are not digested by your body, but help to encourage the development and growth of microbiota in your gut. This is what we want, we want to consume more foods that work this way. Foods that are high in fiber and high in prebiotics. Prebiotics are actually a type of fiber. Probiotics consume prebiotics in your system. Think of them as food that probiotics need to do their job.

You may be interested to know that vegetables, fruits, and whole grains naturally contain prebiotics, but if you really want to get enough on board, you may want to consume foods that have a high content.

Below is a chart of foods that contain high levels of prebiotics:

Evelyn Carmichael

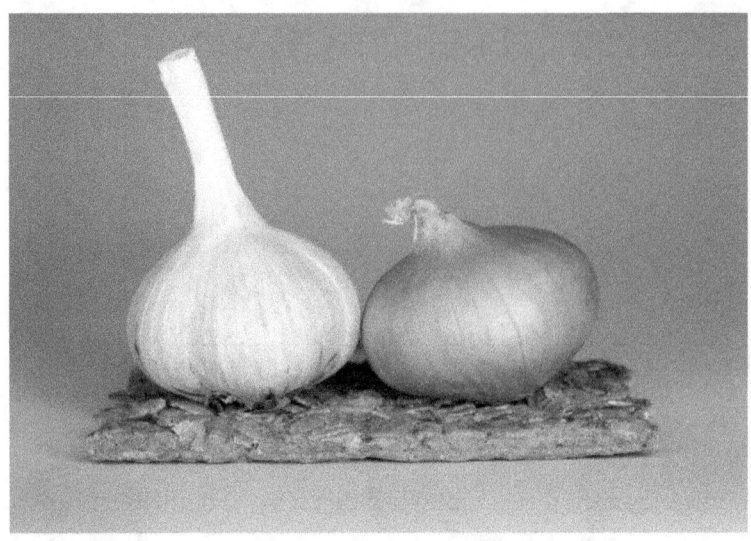

Top Twelve Prebiotic Foods

1. Garlic
2. Onion and Leeks
3. Raw Chicory Root
4. Asparagus
5. Wheat Flour
6. Wheat Bran
7. Banana
8. Dandelion Greens
9. Jerusalem Artichoke
10. Oats
11. Flax and Chia Seeds
12. Apples

✓ Apples – Apples are not only high in fiber, but they also contain a lot of prebiotics. Eaten whole, who chopped up into slices, and enjoyed as a snack or in a smoothie, this fruit will work to improve the health of your gut.

✓ Asparagus (Raw) – Asparagus doesn't just taste great, it is also thought to contain as much as 5% fiber. Some people may find that consuming this vegetable in its raw state is a little difficult, but it can also be enjoyed in smoothies or juices. If you must cook asparagus, please cook it for just a few minutes, so you don't cook out the nutrients.

✓ Bananas – One banana is thought to contain a lot of prebiotics, which means eating just one a day can help to keep your microbiota levels topped up. You can cook the banana if you wish, and include it in your dessert, but the best and most nutritive way is to eat it as it comes, raw!

- ✓ Chicory root – This vegetable has a flavor that's very similar to coffee, which will no doubt be a joy for all coffee lovers to eat.

- ✓ Flax seeds – Flax seeds may be small, but they are also mighty. The work to boost the health of your gut, while also containing fiber.

- ✓ Garlic (Raw) – it is thought that garlic contains many beneficial nutrients, as well as roughly about 17% fiber. Add raw garlic to a wide range of dishes, and enjoy!

- ✓ Jerusalem artichoke – Often called 'Earth apple', Jerusalem artichoke contains 2% fiber, and can be eaten both raw, and cooked. With a wide range of nutritional benefits, this vegetable can help your gut to feel better.

- ✓ Leeks – Containing more nutrients than you probably realize, this vegetable has a delicate onion flavor, and can be eaten in pretty much the same way as onion can. Leeks will help to boost the health of your gut, while also benefiting you in many other ways.

✓ Oats – Oats are not just a great breakfast food, they also come with some good prebiotic benefits. With the ability to improve the health of the bacteria found in your gut, oats can be enjoyed in a wide variety of ways.

✓ Onion (Raw) – onions are high in prebiotics, and can be added to most dishes. The trick is to not over-peel them, as you could be peeling off a lot of the goodness. If raw onions tend to give your heartburn, you may want to think about cooking them instead. They won't contain as many prebiotics if you cook them, but they will still be beneficial.

✓ Wheat bran (Raw) – wheat bran is not only high in fiber, (Roughly 5%), but it can also help to keep your bowels moving. Add wheat bran to yogurts, sprinkle it on top of muffins, or add it to your breakfast cereal, and reap the rewards.

Evelyn Carmichael

CHAPTER 7. PROBIOTICS

Supplements

In addition to eating healthier foods, you should also think about taking some probiotic supplements. Supplements such as these can also help to contribute to the production of healthy microbes in your gut. This is because they work to restore the health of your gut once it has been damaged. Studies have shown that those with a healthy gut probably won't benefit very much from taking these supplements, as they are likely to have all the healthy microbes they need. But it is good to know that if your gut isn't as healthy as it could be, taking a supplement every day can help.

Fermented Foods

Below is a list of foods that contain probiotics in higher amounts to add to your diet.

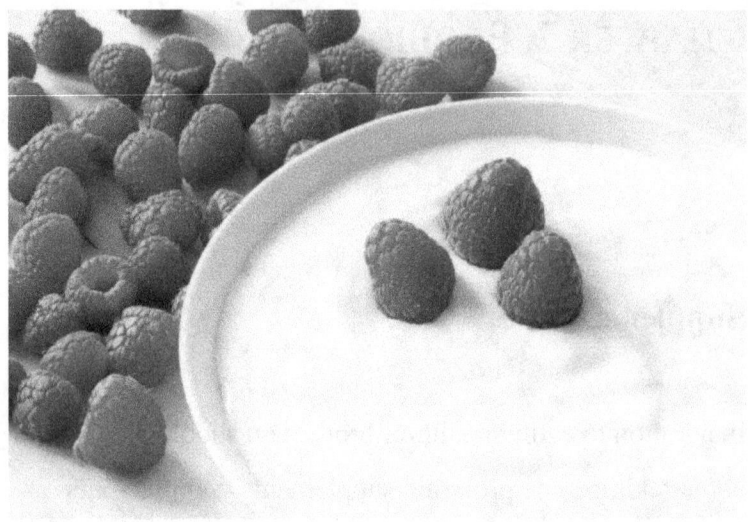

Top Ten Probiotic Foods

1. Yogurt
2. Sour Cream
3. Keifer
4. Raw Cheeses
5. Sauerkraut
6. Dark Chocolate
7. Pickles
8. Kombucha Tea
9. Apple Cider Vinegar
10. Olives (cured)

You will need to be on the lookout for foods that contain probiotics, and many live yogurts and yogurt drinks contain the right cultures needed to restore the balance in your gut. You've probably seen advertisements for small yogurt drinks that are thought to help you get the right balance, but these can often by quite expensive. If you want to save a bit of cash, opt for buying a tub or carton of live yogurt, and have a spoonful or two every day. This will ensure the microbiota in your gut is healthier, and you have more of it too.

Evelyn Carmichael

CHAPTER 8. FOODS AND ENVIRONMENTAL ISSUES THAT CAN CAUSE HARM TO YOUR GUT

Foods to Avoid

If you would like to improve the health of your gut, you should think about eliminating, or cutting down on some of the foods that may be harming your gut. The truth is any food that cause bacteria and or inflammation can lead to poor gut health. Additionally, certain foods may negatively impact the healthy bacteria in your gut or interact in your gut in a way that can cause direct damage to your mucus lining. These foods are:

Sugar

Sugar has certainly received a bad rep in recent years, and rightfully so. Refined sugar can feed the growth of bad bacteria and yeast in your gut causing damage to your mucus lining your gut and ultimately leaky gut. Sugar should only be used sparingly in moderation.

Alcohol

Most of us enjoy a drink now and again, but did you know that alcohol can cause problems in our intestines? It's thought that alcohol consumption can lead to bad bacteria forming in the gut. If you love to drink alcohol, try to replace it with some alcohol-free alternatives, or simply cut down on the amount that you drink.

Artificial sweeteners

Artificial sweeteners aren't that great for the gut, so try to cut these out if you can. I know a lot of people use this type of sweetener because they are trying to reduce their sugar intake, but you won't be doing your gut, or your stomach any favors. Artificial sweeteners can lead to inflammation, which is a known culprit to a leaky gut. New research is also showing that artificial sweeteners can increase microbes that are linked to autoimmune diseases and obesity. If you cannot cut sweeteners out right away, try to cut down a little at a time or use a plant based natural sweetener such as stevia.

Caffeine

I know many people drink a cup of coffee first thing in the morning, but caffeine could be causing a lot more problems than you realize. This is because it can increase stomach acids and affect your adrenal glands. Try to reduce your caffeine intake slowly, before you cut it out altogether.

Evelyn Carmichael

Dairy products

Many of us eat dairy products, but the truth is that we weren't made to. We were only made to consume breast milk, not the multitude of dairy products that you can buy today. A lot of people are lactose intolerant, without even realizing it. For many individuals, dairy causes significant inflammation as well as gas, bloating and other gastrointestinal symptoms.   Do your body a favor, and cut down on the dairy products you consume. Some of the fermented dairy products are good for your health if you can tolerate it (i.e. keifer, yogurt).   You can buy some great substitutes that are highly nutritious and gut healthy. Coconut and Almond milk are high on the list.

Cutting out foods that can harm your gut is the way forward. If you continue to consume the foods that harm you, you will be undoing much of the benefits you receive from the foods that don't do you any harm. Try to cut the harmful foods out slowly but surely, so that you too can feel much better.

Stress

It is easier said than done to eliminate stress from your life. The truth is that stress can cause body wide inflammation, but particularly in the gut. Those feelings of anxiety or stress gurgling up in your stomach is actually doing damage to the lining of your gut. If you are doing all that you can to reduce your stress, take a closer look to how you are able to manage the stress. Some examples of stress relievers are:

- Exercise- making sure you are exercising on a regular basis
- Yoga or Meditation
- Relaxation Breathing
- Therapeutic outlet- art, craft, cooking, or other hobby including exercises such as golf or walking with friends
- Debriefing- if you have a stressful occupation, sometimes just debriefing or talking through a particularly stressful situation is helpful in relieving the stress

- Electronic Breaks- the simple fact of being so tethered to electronic devices is known to cause stress. Schedule electronic free time, but especially in your bedroom and as you are winding down from the day.
- Essential Oils- top oils to relieve stress include rose, lavender, bergamot, chamomile, ylang ylang, and marjoram.

Prescription Medication

While many prescription medications are needed to treat various ailments, please be aware that any medication can change the flora/ bacteria in your gut. You may notice that your symptoms worsen after a dose of antibiotics. An example of this is that women may get a yeast infection after taking a course of antibiotics. Taking extra care of your diet and adding or increasing pre-and probiotics may help decrease this phenomenon when you take medication.

Evelyn Carmichael

CHAPTER 9. TIPS AND TRICKS

This handbook is meant to be an introduction to improving your gut health. Each section could easily fill the content of a book in their own right. However, figuring out the cause or causes that led to poor gut health and changing the way you eat will make a difference.

Don't expect your health to improve right away

It will take time to improve the health of your gut. In fact, it may take months. It all depends on what the health of your gut is like right now, and how hard you work at making those changes. Within a week or two of making changes, you should start to notice a little difference in any heartburn, constipation, bloating, abdominal pain, or diarrhea that you experience, in that the symptoms may not be as bad as they once were. But most physicians would say at least a month is needed to see if the symptoms are truly lessened. You have to remember you are changing a complex ecosystem microrganisms in your gut. It takes time to change the structure of your gut flora and even longer for the healing process to take hold.

Reduce the foods you shouldn't eat slowly but surely

I know how hard it is to change what you eat, but if you take it slowly, and introduce new foods now and again, you will succeed. Don't imagine that it's going to be easy, and accept that you may crave some of the foods you used to love. Take your time, and you're more likely to stick with your new eating plan.

Additionally, take note of removing certain foods and what your symptoms are like. Have they decreased, disappeared, come and go? Make sure you note carefully while you are in a trial and error phase of determining which foods may impact you the most.

Experiment with the new foods you've introduced to your diet

When you introduce a new food to your diet, think about the many ways you can eat it. For example, if you have purchased some whole oats, you can enjoy them as porridge, bake with them, sprinkle them in or on juices and smoothies, and so much more. Foods can be as versatile as you want them to be, so go ahead and experiment.

Realize that everyone is different

What works for someone else might not work for you, and vice versa. While one person might find their gut health has dramatically improved over the period of a month, you may have to wait a bit longer before you see the same results. Everyone is different, and everyone responds to foods in many different ways, so be patient if you need to be, and keep trying to eliminate those nasty symptoms.

Make a note of the meals/snacks that you love

One of the best things that you can do when you change what you eat is to make a note of the meals and snacks that you love. If you make a note of them, you are more likely to enjoy them another time. Making notes like this is a great way for you to stay motivated. Plus, when you are eating new foods, it is important to keep track of how you liked them so you can continue to use them in your diet. Remember, if you go back to eating foods that aren't so good for you, you'll get those nasty symptoms again, and no one wants that.

Don't assume your gut has been permanently 'mended'

It would be nice to think that a few alterations you your diet would result in your gut being completely mended. If you find that your symptoms have improved, you could be forgiven for thinking that you no longer need to think about the health of your gut. It's likely that you will need to keep an eye on what you eat for the rest of your life. Remember that anything you put in to your body that disrupts the gut flora balance can cause damage to your gut lining and trigger inflammation in your body.

Speak to your doctor is you have any concerns

This book is not intended to replace any medical advice or care that a doctor may give you. Neither is it intended to replace any nutritional advice a dietician may give you. If you have any concerns about the health of your gut, please speak to your doctor. You may have an underlying condition that your physician needs to be aware of.

Making the change to your diet slowly but surely can work wonders. After 3-4 weeks, you should start to see a difference in your symptoms. If you continue to eat a better diet, you will continue to feel better in the long term. Having a healthy gut really can make you feel so much better. You will have better digestion, an improved mood, and better overall health. With this is mind it's easy to see why gut health is so important.

Read on for an excerpt of Evelyn Carmichael's book *The Essential Handbook to Lectin*, now on Amazon.

The Essential Handbook to a Healthy Gut

Evelyn Carmichael

THE ESSENTIAL HANDBOOK TO LECTIN

THE PROTEIN CAUSING INFLAMMATION, DIGESTIVE ISSUES, AND WEIGHT GAIN

BY

EVELYN CARMICHAEL

Evelyn Carmichael

INTRODUCTION

Many people eat a gluten-free diet, but they may not be aware that the real culprit that's responsible for their ill health is in fact a protein known as 'Lectin'. This little-known intolerance can cause a wide range of nasty symptoms, from Leaky Gut to Autoimmune Disorders. The good news is that you can help to eliminate those symptoms if you make a few changes to the way that you eat.

If you are one of the thousands of individuals on a gluten free diet but still experiencing the same symptoms that led you to try the diet, you may need to also reduce lectins from your diet. If you did not test positive for a gluten sensitivity, but find you feel a bit better on a gluten free diet, lectin intolerance may also be something you want to consider. Lectins may be responsible for your symptoms and in some cases, may be able to reverse your diagnosis once you decrease them from your diet.

This book will look at exactly what lectins are, the relationship with gluten, and exactly how to reduce them from your diet. With a little bit of guidance and determination, you too may start to feel better by changing the way you eat.

The Essential Handbook to a Healthy Gut

CHAPTER 1. LECTIN AND THE GLUTEN CONNECTION

These days it seems that many individuals are eliminating gluten from their diet. Autoimmune Disease such as Celiac's, Hashimoto's, Rheumatoid Arthritis, and others are on the rise with nearly all individuals trying to reduce inflammation in their body and believe gluten is the culprit. For many, it is, but it may only be one piece in a much larger puzzle.

We know that some people claim to be gluten-intolerant, and state they feel better after eating a gluten-free diet, but there could be another underlying issue that is only partly gluten-related. In fact, the larger and in many cases underlying issue for the diseases themselves is actually something called Lectin.

What is lectin?

Lectin is a protein, and it can be found in plants that need to defend themselves. If you're a keen gardener, or you simply know a little bit about plants, you'll know that plants, like any prey, feel the need to defend themselves from birds, insects, and anything that wants to eat them. Plants contain lectin, which the birds, insects etc. eat, which in turn makes him ill. This is nature's way of defending itself, and telling the birds, insects etc. not to eat them again. Think of lectin as a low-level toxin that the plant uses to make its prey not want to touch it again.

The fact of the matter is that when we decide to eat these plants, we're not as immune to the lectin as we might like to think we are. When many of us eat plants that contain lectin, we can start to feel unwell, perhaps we take an indigestion tablet, or a painkiller to help combat our symptoms, without realizing what is actually going on.

So, one could just give up plant based foods in their diet, right? Unfortunately, lectins are found in every living thing. In fact, this protein is found in animal based products as well. Newer research shows that dairy products have the highest levels of lectin of all animal based foods. Fruits and vegetables are also not immune, as well as legumes, spices, oils, nuts, seeds, and sweeteners. This makes giving up Lectin entirely an impossible task. To make matters worse, exact lectin content is largely unknown per specific food as this protein occurs naturally and his highly individualized. There are general ideas on high versus low lectin foods that can assist you in significantly decreasing your Lectin intake.

The Science Behind Lectin

Lectins are a carbohydrate-binding protein that can attach to cell membranes. They become the 'communicator' for cells to organize and connect with their environment. There are several different types of lectins in various living organisms. In plants, lectins are primarily found in the roots and seeds, with the lowest level of lectin found in the leaves.

There are thousands of different types of lectins, many that have not been studied. Of those that have had the most research, 13 major classifications of lectin have emerged and their functions vary slightly, but two classes, agglutinins and prolamins, appear to cause the most damage to our bodies and are found in high lectin foods. Agglutinins and prolamins can have a major impact in how our gut and immune system functions often causing an inflammatory response.

When your intestinal wall is permeated or damaged by lectins, the protein leaks out into your bloodstream. At that time, the lectin can bind to glycoproteins that are found on the surface of most cells as well as to antibodies. The cells can be located anywhere in your body, including your joints, brain, liver, heart, and kidneys. Your body responds by attacking those cells which contains healthy material underneath. This triggering is known as an autoimmune response. Continual responses can lead to autoimmune diseases.

Where does gluten fit into all this?

You may now be wondering where gluten fits into all this, and you may be surprised to know that gluten is thought to be a type of lectin, specifically belonging to the Prolamin class. This potentially means that while you're cutting gluten out of your diet, you're not actually resolving the issue. This is because other foods can contain lectin, not just those that also contain gluten. What this means is that even though you're cutting gluten out of your diet, you're perhaps not doing as much as you can to combat those nasty symptoms you suffer from. This may be why many people who have a gluten sensitivity who cut gluten from their diet still have symptoms, albeit to a lesser degree.

Some of the highest lectin level foods contain gluten such as grains.

To find out more about Lectins and how they impact your health, please visit https://www.amazon.com/Essential-Handbook-Lectin-Inflammation-Digestive-ebook/dp/B072363VMQ/.

Evelyn Carmichael

ABOUT THE AUTHOR

Evelyn Carmichael

Evelyn was in the world of corporate finance before switching her life path after a successful battle with breast cancer. She is a personal life coach, fitness guru, and healthy lifestyle advocate.

Find out more on Facebook or at
https://www.amazon.com/Evelyn-Carmichael/e/B01MQYHZLC

Evelyn Carmichael

OTHER BOOKS BY EVELYN CARMICHAEL

Evelyn is the author of the Essential Handbook Series.

Her titles include the following:

The Essential Handbook to High Fiber Diet

The Essential Handbook to Paleo Instant Pot Cooking

The Essential Handbook to Lectin

The Essential Handbook to the Alzheimer's Diet

The Essential Handbook to Superfood Smoothies

The Essential Handbook to Hashimoto's

The Essential Handbook to Herbal Remedies

The Essential Handbook to Hygge

The Essential Handbook to Diabetic Instant Pot Cooking

Evelyn Carmichael

The Essential Handbook to Gluten Free Instant Pot Cooking

The Essential Handbook to Avocados The Superfood that Reduce Inflammation and lowers blood sugar, blood pressure, and your cholesterol

The Essential Handbook to Reversing Prediabetes and Diabetes: Meal Plans and Recipes to Reduce Your Blood Sugar Levels and Eliminate Diabetes and Prediabetes

The Essential Handbook to Turmeric and Ginger: The Anti-Inflammatory Duo that will Change your Life

The Essential Handbook to Coconut Oil: Tips, Recipes, and How to use for weight loss and in your daily life

The Essential Handbook to Apple Cider Vinegar: Tips and Recipes for Weight Loss and Improving your Health, Beauty, & Home

The Art of Keeping Goals

The Essential Handbook for Choosing the Right Diet: A Guide to the Most Popular Diets and if They are Right for You

The Essential Handbook to Natural Living

The Essential Handbook to Essential Oils: Tips and Recipes for Weight Loss, Stress Relief, and Pain Management

Knee Supports: Uses, Exercises, and Benefits

Evelyn Carmichael

AUTHOR NOTE

If you enjoyed this book, found it useful or otherwise then I'd really appreciate it if you would post a short review on Amazon. I do read all the reviews personally so that I can continually write what people are wanting.

Thanks for your support!

Evelyn Carmichael